SOY

Asia's Hidden Healer

Deanne Tenney

WOODLAND PUBLISHING
Pleasant Grove, UT

TABLE OF CONTENTS

SOY

INTRODUCTION

In recent years, the focus of the natural health community has been placed squarely on phytochemicals, which are naturally occurring chemicals that have the ability to protect the body against disease. Some are thought to lower cholesterol, some fortify cancer defenses, and others work as powerful antioxidants.

Soy is one of the richest sources of these phytochemicals found anywhere. Soybeans are packed full of these powerful compounds and researchers are tirelessly exploring the myriad of positive health benefits soy may offer.

Many individuals, however, have resisted adapting their diets to include more soy. The flavor of soy is unusual to those in the Western world; basically, we are just not used to the taste and texture of soy-based products. In addition, most of the soy products in the United States have been traditionally used to feed farm animals.

But the trend is slowly shifting. The health benefits of this remarkable—and naturally-occuring—compound cannot be denied. In fact, an increase of soy in the diet may dramatically reduce the risk of two of the most dreaded diseases that can strike down every human being: heart disease and cancer.

The Asian Connection

Those who inhabit the Japanese islands have the longest life expectancy in the world. They also have a much smaller risk for breask, colon, prostate, and lung cancer. And heart disease is minimal, at best. Not coincidentally, the Japanese also consume much higher amounts of soy than any other populace in the world.

While the U.S. dutifully grows the most soy in the world, more than half of it is shipped to other nations and the other half is gobbled up by farm animals. Essentially, there are massive amounts of soy that are readily available to those in this country who are interested in adding it to the diet along with other wholesome and healthy foods. If the Japanese are any indicator, soy consumption may be the key to a longer and healthier life.

THE HISTORY OF SOY

Soybeans have been eaten for thousands of years by both humans and animals. Areas of northern China are credited with first cultivating soybeans for consumption before recorded history, more than 13,000 years ago. Over the centuries, travellers and migrating groups of Chinese spread the soybean plant throughout Asia. The Chinese highly revere the soybean and consider it to be one of their five sacred grains, along with rice, barley, wheat and millet.[1] In fact, the Chinese so admire the effects of soy that it was highly recommended in the *Chinese Materia Medica*, a rare honor indeed. In the past, it has even been used to treat various conditions such as renal disease, edema, skin disease, constipation, anemia and diarrhea.[2]

Soybeans were carted to Japan from China sometime during the seventh century. The introduction of soybeans to Europe is thought to have been by Kaempfer, a German botanist, in the 17th century.[3]

Sometime during the 1800s, soybeans made their way to the United States aboard a trade ship from China. Even so, there was little interest in the soybean until the early 1900s. In 1930, the manufacturers of cooking oil became interested in the use of the soybean for oil. Varieties of soybean oil have been improved over the years, with specific emphasis being placed on higher yields and oil content. Interestingly, the United States is the world's leading soybean producer,[4] with more than 50 percent of the world's legumes grown on American soil. As a result, the soybean is the most financially productive crop in the United States.

NUTRIENTS IN SOYBEANS

The soybean is one of the most valuable foods known to man. An acre of soybeans can produce 20 times more protein than beef;[5] there are few, if any, plants that compare with the soybean in regard to total nutritional value. Soybeans contain important vitamins and minerals including calcium, phosphorus, iron, zinc, vitamin E, and B-complex vitamins. When compared to other legumes, the soybean is higher in essential fatty acids and lower in carbohydrate content. Soy also provides every amino acid necessary to manufacture protein in the body. Without a doubt, soy is an incredible source of valuable nutrients.

Protein

Protein in soybeans is comparable to the protein in animal-based products—beef, chicken, etc. All the amino acids necessary to make protein (there are 20 amino acids that are vital to maintain human life). One drawback, though: soy contains lower-than-needed levels of methionine, an amino acid that is found in grains like wheat and yeast. When soy is combined with other grains, the building blocks that comprise every human protein are complete.

Fiber

The health advantages of soy fiber have been thoroughly researched and documented in clinical studies. Of the fiber that is found in soybeans, 94 percent of it is insoluble (just six percent is soluble.)

Phytate

For years, this stored form of phosphorous was believed to be an "anti-nutrient"—a negative tag applied to things like white sugar. Recently, however, phytate has been found to play a role in disease prevention. Phytate is a powerful antioxidant and may play a significant role in preventing cancer and heart disease.

Omega-3 Essential Fatty Acids

These acids, found in soy oil, are a form of healthy fats with multiple properties that improve health. The total fat content of soybeans is about 18 percent, a little higher, perhaps, than most health-conscious people would like. But, 85 percent of the fat in soybeans is of the harmless unsaturated variety, and just 15 percent is saturated.[6]

Protease Inhibitors

Protease inhibitors are phytochemicals that used to be considered detrimental to the health. Research has found that protease inhibitor can actually aid in inhibiting cancers of the skin, bladder, colon, lungs, pancreas, mouth, and esophagus. Protease inhibitors work to block the activity of proteases, which are enzymes, that may encourage tumor growth. Protease inhibitors may also protect against the harm caused by radiation and free radical damage.

Phytosterols

Phytosterols are similar in structure to the cholesterols found in plants. They compete with dietary cholesterol for absorption in the colon which means that less cholesterol is being absorbed into the colon and more passes out with every bowel movement; essentially, the phytosterols block the cholesterol absorption sites. Phytosterols also aid in cancer and ulcer prevention, particularly in the colon, where they neutralize the damage caused by bile acids.

Saponins

Saponins are naturally occurring substances in soybeans

and other foods that reduce the growth and development of colon and melanoma cancer cells.

Isoflavones

Isoflavones are unique to soybeans. They are very similar to estrogen, but less powerful. They aid in the prevention of breast cancer by connecting to estrogen receptors on tissue cells that may become carcinogenic with potent levels of estrogen. Isoflavones do not restrict the positive activity of estrogen but reduce its cancer-causing potential. Asian women and vegetarians who consume soy have very low incidence of breast cancer. Isoflavones not only help prevent cancer but can assist in preventing heart disease by lowering cholesterol levels.

Genistein

Genistein is the main isoflavone in soybeans. It is one of the most powerful flavonoids discovered to date. Clinical studies have found that the genistein in soy to be a powerful tool in cancer prevention and treatment. There have been over 200 separate research papers written on genistein since 1986. Some consider it to be one of the most powerful anti-cancer agents anywhere in the world. It works by regulating the action of some enzymes that are involved in the cancer process. One of the most amazing aspects of genistein is that is able to physically alter cancerous cells and neutralize their danger by turning them into normal, harmless cells. It also inhibits the growth of blood vessels that feed the cancer, depriving the malignant cells of nutrients. Genistein is also a powerful antioxidant that minimizes free radical damage known to cause cancer and other diseases.[7]

Daidzein

Yet another antioxidant flavonoid found in soybeans is daidzein. When daidzein is broken down by the body, it results in ipriflavone, which is currently under investigation for its role in preventing osteoporosis.[8] Daidzein may also be helpful in inhibiting the growth of cancer cells.

CARDIOVASCULAR DISEASE AND SOY

Heart disease is the leading cause of death in most developed countries. And in countries that are shaking off the shackles of undeveloped squalor, heart disease occurence is drastically rising as people adapt Western eating and lifestyle habits. But cultures where soybeans are consumed regularly have been found to have much lower incidence of heart disease as well as lower occurences of other fatal conditions like various forms of cancer, liver disease, etc. In Japan, the modern society that consumes more soybeans than any other, deaths caused by heart disease are rare—nearly one-half of the rate in the United States.

With heart disease as widespread and common as it is, perplexed physicians prescribe cholesterol-lowering drugs to their patients. But drug therapy is incredibly expensive and there are adverse effects. Moreover, cholesterol-lowering drugs may not even mean a longer life for the patient.

As a result, it may be prudent for medical professionals to look at natural methods of lowering cholesterol and preventing cardiovascular disease. Clinical studies have discovered that soy protein can actually be useful in lowering cholesterol levels. Interestingly, many physicians don't have any idea about soy and its potentially life-saving attributes.

At the First International Symposium on Soy and Chronic Diseases held in Phoenix in 1994, a paper was presented by Cesare Sirtori, M.D., a professor of clinical pharmacology at the University of Milan in Italy. Sirtori's paper discussed the benefits of soy food in helping to cut cholesterol. Volunteers with very high levels of cholesterol (at least 353 mg/dl) were recruited for the study and were separated into two groups. One group continued eating a low-fat diet while the other added soy to their diets. After a four-week trial period, the group on the diet without soy had the same cholesterol levels while the group of soy eaters had reduced their cholesterol levels and average of 27 percent.[9]

Resultingly, it was determined that soy lowered LDL cholesterol (bad cholesterol), and even raised the levels of HDL cholesterol (good cholesterol).

Soy-based products may work by increasing the activity of LDL receptors, which grab deposits of LDL and deliver it to the liver where it is broken down and excreted from the body. Soy contains a variety of phytoestrogens that may be responsible for this activity. Soy may also be effective in that it prevents cholesterol from sticking to the artery walls, which, of course, is the precursor to more serious heart problems.

James W. Anderson lead a team of researchers from the University of Kentucky at Lexington in analyzing the results of 38 controlled trials to determine the effects of soy protein and a reduction of cholesterol in humans. There were more than 740 individuals involved in the various studies. The average amount of soy consumed was 47 grams per day. The results were significant. When soy protein was eaten instead of animal-based protein, serum concentrations of LDL cholesterol and equally dangerous triglycerides actually thinned out.

The reduction in LDL cholesterol was the greatest in subjects with the highest initial serum cholesterol concentrations. But even individuals with initial serum cholesterol levels below 200 mg/dl had an estimated decrease of 7.7 percent.[10] The results of this study were compiled from a series of small trials and then grouped together statistically. As a result, many skeptics claim that the data is irrelevant. But further studies have provided more information regarding the cholesterol-killing benefits associated with soy consumption.

Italy has long been a center of study on soy protein and its beneficial effects on the body. Researchers in Italy have consistently seen reductions in LDL levels around 22 to 25 percent. Those with the highest initial levels showed the greatest reduction. Casare R. Sirtori suggested that soy may only work significantly for those with cholesterol levels above 240 mg/dl.[11]

Studies have also found that cholesterol can be reduced as well in individuals with normal cholesterol levels. A clinical study conducted by K.K. Carroll at the University of Western Ontario followed the blood cholesterol of women with normal levels. These women were divided into two categories. The first ate a well-balanced diet containing both animal and plant protein sources. The second group was placed on a diet with soy protein derived from soy sources. The cholesterol levels of the women on the soy diet dropped by about five percent. The other group remained the same.[12]

These conclusive and irrevocable studies and their findings should motivate physicians and dieticians to recommend the use of soy protein in the diets of their patients with high cholesterol levels.

CANCER & OTHER AILMENTS

Evidence is everywhere that legitimizes the anticancer potential of soybeans. In fact, soybeans contain at least five different known anticarcinogens including protease inhibitors, phytates, phytosterols, saponins, phenolic acids, and isoflavones. Isoflavones, in particular, have gained considerable recognition for their effects in treating and preventing a wide array of cancers, including those that attack the lungs, breasts, the colon, prostate, skin, and liver.[13]

An article in the *Journal of Nutrition*, March 1995, suggests the use of soybeans for cancer prevention in many different organ systems. A diet high in soy products is recommended because of the positive results of animal studies involving soy intake.[14]

Asian countries including China, Japan, Korea, and Thailand have much lower death rates from cancer than Western nations. Individuals living in some Western countries have ten times the risk of developing cancer as individuals living in Asian nations. Studies seem to point to soy as a contributing component to cancer prevention when comparing Asian and Western eating habits.

There are hundreds of studies completed and many more in progress punctuating the benefits of a soy-based diet, including its role in cancer prevention. Soy is something that should not be overlooked for health and vitality.

Breast Cancer

Breast cancer is a condition that affects a growing number of women in Western nations. The incidence is much greater in the West than in Asian countries such as Japan, China,

Thailand, and Korea. Intrigued by the wide gap between the rates of breast cancer, many researchers have conducted studies that have seemingly uncovered a major causal factor: the consumption of soy-based products. In Asian nations, people consume much higher levels of soy than those in the West.

Kenneth Setchell, Ph.D., a professor of pediatrics at the Children's Hospital Medical Center in Cincinnati, found a correlation between soy intake and longer menstrual cycles. Six women in their twenties were given two ounces of TVP (a soy product) in addition to their regular diet. Their menstrual cycles increased by two to five days. A longer menstrual cycle means there is less exposure to estrogen for women. Researchers believe that lower levels of estrogen exposure means a smaller risk for developing breast cancer. Asian women generally have longer menstrual cycles and lower risk of breast cancer than Western women. When miso (a stronger soy-based product) was substituted for TVP, an even greater effect was seen.[15] Adding soy to the diet may lessen the number of menstrual periods a woman experiences over a lifetime reducing exposure to estrogen.

Dietary estrogens such as genistein contribute in the prevention of hormone-dependent cancers. The action of genistein in soy products is similar to that of Tamoxifen, a prescribed drug often used to prevent a recurrence of breast cancer.

Another study researched the hormonal status and menstrual cycle length in six premenopausal women with regular menstrual cycles. They were each given 60 grams of soy protein each day containing 45 mg of isoflavones. After one month, their cycles were longer and menstruation was delayed. A similar reaction is seen with Tamoxifen, which is used in treating breast cancer.[17]

Prostate cancer

Prostate cancer is becoming an increasingly serious problem among men in many Western cultures. It is the second most common type of cancer among men (skin cancer is first). Contrastingly, a low mortality rate from prostate cancer has been found in many Asian cultures with diets high in soybean products.

Prostate cancer is among the cancers known to be hormone-sensitive—that is, hormones such as testosterone and estrogen fuel their growth.

A smaller ratio of Japanese men die from prostate cancer than in any other society in the world. One study followed a group of Japanese men eating a low-fat diet rich in soy products as compared to a group of Finnish men. The isoflavone levels in the Japanese men were seven to ten times higher than in the Finnish men. The assumption is that the higher levels of soy in the diet of the Japanese men contribute to lower rates of prostate cancer cell growth.[18]

A study undertaken in 1989 involved 8,000 Hawaiian men of Japanese ancestry over a period of twenty years. The men who consumed the highest amounts of tofu in their diets had the lowest rates of prostate cancer. (Tofu is high in soy protein and protective isoflavones.)[19]

Colon Cancer

Charles Poole, Ph.D., a Harvard researcher, found a correlation between high soy consumption and a decrease in colon cancer risk.[20] Americans who consumed soybeans and tofu regularly had a significantly lower risk of developing colon cancer. Individuals who eat high soy diets tend to eat less meat, which may also be a factor in a lower incidence of cancer in the bowels.

Menopausal Problems

Menopause is dreaded by many women, who will unavoidably have to deal with it at some point in their lives. Menopause refers to the end of the menstrual cycle with the cessation of ovulation and menstrual periods. This period could take months or even years to complete. Some women have serious problems associated with menopause such as hot flashes, vaginal dryness, sweating, headaches, irregular periods, and heart palpitations. A few women seem to go through the change with little or no complications.

Asian women generally have fewer problems going through menopause than Western women. One Japanese study published in the *Lancet* found a correlation between a high soy diet and very few physical and mental complaints as women begin menopause.[21] The estrogen-like components in soy are thought to act like hormonal estrogen preventing menopausal problems. Symptoms such as hot flashes, dysfunctional uterine bleeding, vaginal dryness and mood swings are rare among menopausal women in Japan. It is felt by some researchers that the addition of soy in the diet could reduce or even replace the need for hormone replacement therapy.[22]

A recent study by a group of Canadian researchers of the correlation of Japanese women and menopause reported that "the hot flush or flash, seen in the West as the sine qua non of the menopausal woman, were mentioned by only 12 of the 105 women and no one talked about night sweats."

In another study, researchers compared the menopausal experiences of Japanese, Canadian, and U.S. women. The Japanese women had far fewer physical complaints than did the Western women. Nearly 35 percent of the U.S. women and 31 percent of the Canadian women reported having hot flashes, versus only 12.4 percent of the Japanese women. More than 38.1 percent of the American women complained of a lack of energy; only 6 percent of the Japanese women. More than 35 percent of the U.S. women complained of depression, only 10.3 of the Japanese said they felt depressed. In fact, researchers reported that few Japanese women were on any medication (hormone replacement therapy) for menopause. However, Japanese women did use more herbs and herbal teas.[23]

Osteoporosis

Osteoporosis is a condition most often found in women after menopause. Bones affected by osteoporosis become thin and porous. The most common sites of problems involve the spine, hips and ribs.

Soy products may aid in the prevention of osteoporosis. They are an excellent source of the minerals boron and calcium. One study conducted at the University of Texas Health Sciences Center found that volunteers in the study excreted 50 percent less calcium in their urine when they replaced animal products (meats, milk, etc.) with soy-based products.[24]

A study done to determine the future problems of osteoporosis in Asian women found that rural populations have less of a risk because of their diets high in protective foods such as bioflavonoids and phytoestrogen-rich foods such as soybeans.[25] Asian researchers were concerned with an aging population in their countries and predicted an increase in problems associated with osteoporosis. But studies found that because of the rich-in-soy diet of rural Asian women, their risk of developing osteoporosis was relatively low when compared with women in Western civilizations.

Diabetes

Diabetes is serious condition common in Western civilizations. As with some other serious diseases, diabetes is relatively rare in Asian cultures. Some attribute this to the fiber content in soybeans. Some forms of fiber, including soy fiber, have been found to help control blood glucose levels, which are erratic at best in diabetics.[26]

The phytates found in soybeans may also help protect the body, working as an antioxidant against free radical damage. Diabetes may be precipitated by free radical damage, and soybeans may help protect from this condition.

Diarrhea

Diarrhea can be a serious problem for infants and young children who can easily become dehydrated. One study conducted at the University of Nebraska College of Medicine found that soy fiber helped to reduce the duration of diarrhea caused by bacterial and viral sources. A randomized, blinded clinical trial was conducted with American children fed either soy formula or soy fiber supplemented formula. Infants over six months of age were fed formula supplemented with soy fiber. They showed a significantly shorter duration of diarrhea—9.7 hours as compared to 23.1 hours.[27]

SOY PRODUCTS

Soybeans can be used in many forms. The whole bean can be cooked or sprouted and added to recipes. They can be substituted for other legumes or grains in soups, casseroles, etc. Soy is a high quality and beneficial form of protein.

TOFU: Tofu is probably the most popular of all forms of soy. It is mild tasting with a cheese-like consistency. Tofu or bean curd is often used as a meat substitute. It is made by curdling soy milk, discarding the whey, and pressed into a cake form. The amount of pressing determines the texture of the tofu. It is very mild and absorbs the flavor of the food it is cooked with. Tofu is often used as a cheese substitute for those sensitive to dairy products. Tofu can be purchased in different forms: firm tofu, silken tofu, yakidofu, and koyodofu.

MISO: Miso is a fermented soybean paste often used for seasoning and in soups. It is made by combining soybeans, salt, and water with a cultured grain. The product is then aged in cedar vats for as long as three years. The strong, robust flavor makes it great for seasoning. Many beneficial affects are associated with miso consumption.

NATTO: Natto is a bacterially fermented form of soybean. Whole cooked soybeans are added to a bacillus nato culture, forming a sticky coating. Natto has a strong smell and cheeselike texture. It is used as a spread or in soups. The whole soybean is used.

TEMPEH: Tempeh is made from mold fermented soybeans. The beans are soaked overnight and then cooked until soft. A mold is added to the cooked soybeans and then the mixture sits for 24 hours. It is often pressed into a patty or cake, marinated and grilled or baked. Tempeh has a nutty, smoky flavor and the texture is similar to meat.

TAMARI: Tamari is a naturally fermented soy sauce.

SOY FLOUR: Soy flour is very high in protein, and can be combined with other flours to increase protein. Eggs can be replaced in recipes with one tablespoon of soy flour and two tablespoons of water for each egg.

SOY MILK: Soy milk is made from pureed soybeans in water. This creamy beverage is made by soaking and grinding whole soybeans in water. Soy milk is lactose free and is often used as a substitute for those who suffer from lactose intolerance. It is made to taste similar to milk and can be purchased in a variety of flavors in health food stores and supermarkets. Soy milk is growing in popularity as it becomes more available.

SOY OIL: Soy oil is extracted from the soybean. It is a light, bland oil often used for cooking. It is a common ingredient in processed foods, baked goods and salad dressings. Soy oil is rich in omega-3 and omega-6 fatty acids which are beneficial for health.

SOY SPROUTS: Soy sprouts can be added to salads, sandwiches or other dishes.

SOY GRITS: After soy oil is extracted from the beans, what is left is ground and compressed into soy grits.

SOY BURGER: This is a meat substitute patty usually sold frozen at the supermarket.

SAFETY OF SOY PRODUCTS

Soy has been used for thousands of years, and such a long history generally means it is safe. There are some individuals who may be sensitive to soy protein just as some have allergies to eggs, wheat and dairy products.

"SOY GOOD" RECIPES

Blueberry and Soy Muffins

1 1/2 cup whole wheat pastry flour
1 cup soy flour
2 t. baking powder
1/2 t. salt
1/2 cup maple syrup
1/3 cup soft silken tofu
3/4 cup soy milk
3 T. canola oil
1/2 cup fresh or frozen (thawed) blueberries
Combine flour, baking powder and salt. In blender combine maple syrup, tofu, soy milk and oil until smooth.

Combine ingredients and fold in blueberries. Fill 12 greased muffins tins 2/3 full. Bake and 375° for approximately 25 minutes.

Breakfast Strawberry and Soy Drink

1 medium banana sliced
1 cup fresh or frozen (thawed) strawberries
1 1/2 cup soy milk
1 T. orange juice concentrate
1 t. honey
1/4 cup cold water and 4 ice cubes
Combine all ingredients in a blender and blend until smooth.

Tofu Smoothie

1 package soft tofu
1 cup orange juice
1 t. lemon juice
1 cup strawberries
2 t. honey
10 ice cubes
Combine all ingredients in a blender until smooth.

Eggless Egg Salad

1 pound tofu
2 T. soy sauce
1 t. mustard
2 T. reduced fat mayonnaise
4 T. fat free sour cream
2 celery stalks, chopped

2 T. minced onions
2 T. honey
1 T. lemon juice
1/2 t. garlic powder
salt and pepper to taste
Mash the tofu and combine with other ingredients. Serve on bread, cracker, biscuits or as a dip.

Tofu/Cheese Spread

1/2 cup cheddar cheese, grated
1/2 cup Parmesan cheese, grated
1/2 cup tofu, mashed
1/2 cup mayonnaise
3 t. onion grated
1 t. curry powder
Mix together and serve on crackers or bread.

Tofu Vegetable Salad

2 cups sliced tomatoes
2 cups sliced cucumbers
2 cups sliced celery
1 green pepper chopped
1 cup sliced mushrooms
1/2 large onion chopped
1/2 cup chopped fresh parsley
Mix together the above with dressing below.

Dressing

1/2 pound drained tofu, mash thoroughly
2 T. lime juice

3 T. olive oil
1/2 t. salt
1 clove garlic minced
Blend until smooth and mix with vegetable salad.

Tofu Stir-Fry

1 pound firm tofu cut in 1/2 inch squares
1/4 cup soy sauce
1 1/2 T. cornstarch
2 T. canola oil
1 pound broccoli, washed and chopped
1 onion, chopped
2 celery stalks, sliced
2 garlic cloves, chopped
1 cup bean sprouts

Marinate the tofu in 2 T. soy sauce for 10 to 15 minutes. (Light soy sauce may be substituted) Mix the remaining soy sauce and cornstarch together. Stir fry the tofu in a skillet or wok until light brown. Remove the tofu and stir fry the broccoli, onions, celery and garlic for 3 to 5 minutes. Add the bean sprouts and continue cooking for 1 more minute. Serve over cooked brown rice.

Tofu Quiche

2 t. canola oil
1 onion, minced
2 cups mushrooms, sliced
1/4 t. salt
4 eggs well beaten
1/2 cup soy milk

1 (10 1/2 ounce) package of firm tofu
4 ounces Swiss or sharp cheddar cheese
Blend eggs, milk and tofu in a blender until smooth. Combine other ingredients and stir well. Spray a 10 inch quiche dish and pour mixture into the dish. Bake at 350° for approximately 40 minutes or until set.

Soybean and Bulgur Casserole

1/2 c. dried soybeans
1 cup bulgur wheat
1 cup boiling water
2 T. olive oil
1 onion, chopped
1 quart tomatoes
1 green pepper, chopped
2 cups feta cheese, crumbled
1 t. cumin
1/2 t. cayenne pepper
2 T. parsley, minced
salt and pepper to taste

Soak soybeans in water and cover overnight. Drain and put beans in a blender and add one cup water. Blend until smooth. Pour 1 cup boiling water over bulgur and set aside. Preheat oven to 350°. Heat oil in a skillet and saute onion and green pepper until tender. Add soybeans, then bulgur, salt, pepper, cayenne and parsley. Oil a three quart casserole dish and spread half the mixture in the bottom, and sprinkle with half the cheese. Combine the tomatoes, cumin and spread over the cheese. Repeat the mixture, cheese and tomatoes. Cover and bake for approximately one hour.

Tofu and Vegetable Soup

1 package (10 1/2 ounces) soft tofu
2 T. olive oil
1 onion, chopped
2 garlic clove, minced
3 celery stalks, chopped
3 carrots, chopped
2 cups cabbage, chopped
1 large can tomatoes
2 cups cooked whole grain pasta
4 cups chicken broth
2 T. fresh parsley, chopped
2 T. fresh dill, chopped
salt and pepper to taste

Heat the olive oil and add onions and garlic. Saute for 3 minutes. Add celery, carrots and cabbage and continue to saute for another few minutes. Add the other ingredients except the tofu. Blend the tofu in the blender and slowly add to the soup. Heat and serve.

Tofu Potato Soup

3 cups potatoes, peeled and cubed
1/2 cup carrots, sliced
2 stalks celery, sliced
1 medium onion, chopped
2 cloves garlic, minced
2 T. olive oil
2 cups chicken broth
2 cups water

1 package soft tofu
seasonings to taste
Heat olive oil in skillet and add onions and garlic. Cook
for 2 to 3 minutes. In a pot combine other ingredients,
except tofu, season and bring to a boil. Simmer on low heat
for one hour. Blend tofu in a blender and slowly add to soup.
Reheat and serve.

ENDNOTES

1. The 1995 Grolier Multimedia Encyclopedia, (Danbury, CT: Grolier Electronic Publishing, Inc., 1995), 1.
2. Stephen Holt, M.D., Soya For Health, (Larchmont, N.Y.: Mary Ann Liebert, Inc., 1996) 3.
3. Frank Murray, "Is Genistein the Key to Soy's Success?," Let's Live, August, 1996, 54.
4. Grolier Multimedia Encyclopedia, 1995 (1).
5. Michael T. Murray, The Healing Power of Foods, (Rocklin, CA: Prima Publishing, 1993) 168.
6. Michael Murray, 169.
7. Mark Messina and Virginia Messina, The Simple Soybean And Your Health, (New York: Avery Publishing Group, 1994).
8. Rona P. Zoltan, MD.., "The Joys of Soy," Health Naturally, October/November 1997, 23.
9. Michael Castleman, The Healing Herbs, (Emmaus, Pennsylvania: Rodale Press, Inc., 1996) 174-75.
10. James. W. Anderson, BM Johnstone, ME Cook-Newell, "Meta-analysis of the effects of soy protein intake on serum lipids," New England Journal of Medicine, (88) (1993): 3008-29.
11. Kristine Napier, "Taking Soy to Heart," Harvard Health Letter, November 1995, 2.
12. K.K. Carroll, "Review of clinical studies on cholesterol-lowering response to soy protein," Journal of ther American Dietetic Association, 91 (1991)d 820-7.
13. Murray, 54.
14. A. R. Kennedy, "The evidence for soybean products as cancer preventive agents," Journal of Nutrition, 125 (2) (February 1995) 733S-743S.
15. Kenneth Setchell, S.P. Borriello, P. Hulme, M. Axelson, "Nonsteroidal estrogens of dietary origin: Possible roles in hormone-dependent disease, American Journal of Clinical Nutrition 40 (1984): 569-78.

16. B.A. Stoll, "Eating to beat breast cancer: potential role for soy supplements," Ann Oncol 8 (3) (March 1997) 223-25.

17. A. Cassidy, S. Bingham, K. Setchell, "Biological effects of soy protein rich in isoflavones on menstrual cycle of premenopausal women," American Journal of Clinical Nutrition 60 (3) (Sept. 1994): 151-3.

18. H. Adlercreutz, H. Markkanen, S. Watanabe, "Plasma concentrations of phyto-oestrogens in Japanese men," Lancet 342 (8881) (Nov., 13, 1993) 1209-1210.

19. R. K. Severson, A. Nomura, J.S. Grove, G.N. Stemmermann, "A prospective study of demographics, diet and prostate cancer among men of Japanese ancestry in Hawaii," Cancer Research 9 (1989): 1857-60.

20. Michael Castleman, Nature's Cures, (Emmaus, Pennsylania: Rodale Press, Inc. 1996) 175.

21. H. Aldercreutz, E. Hamalaiene, S. Gorbach, and B. Goldin, "Dietary phyto-oestrogenletter and the menopause in Japan," Lancet, 339 (1992): 1233.

22. Zoltan, 23

23. Earl Mindell, Earl Mindell's Soy Miracle, (New York: Fireside, 1995) 74.

24. Susan Smith Jones and Brian Bailey, ÒTofu is a Superfood for the 1990's," Let's Live, June 1995, 84.

25. P.C. Kao and F.K. P'eng, "How to reduce the risk factors of osteoporosis in Asia," Chung Hua I Hsueh Tsa Chih (Taipei), 55 (3), (March 1995) 209-13.

26. D.J. Jenkins, D.V. Goff, A.R. Leeds, K.G. Alberti, T.M. Wolever, M.A. Gassull, and T.D. Hockaday, ÒUnabsorbable carbohydrates and diabetes: Decreased post-prandial hyperglycaemia," Lancet, 24 (2) (July 1976) 172-4.

27. J.A. Vanderhoof, N.D. Murray, C.L. Paule, and K.M. Ostrom, "Use of soy fiber in acute diarrhea in infants and toddlers," Clinical Pedicatrics, 36 (3), (March 1997) 135-9.